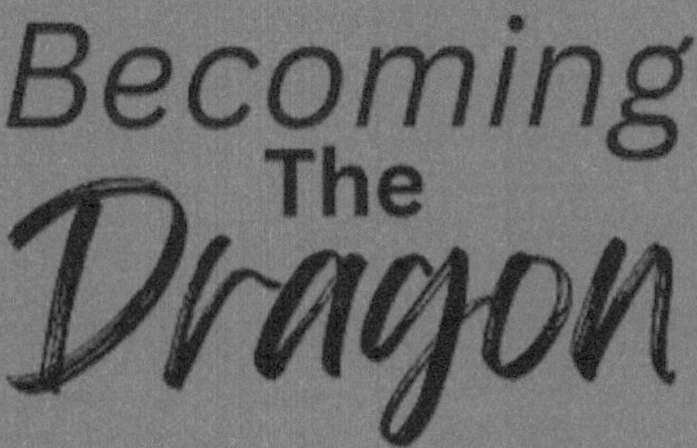

The Beginners Guide to Quick Fitness

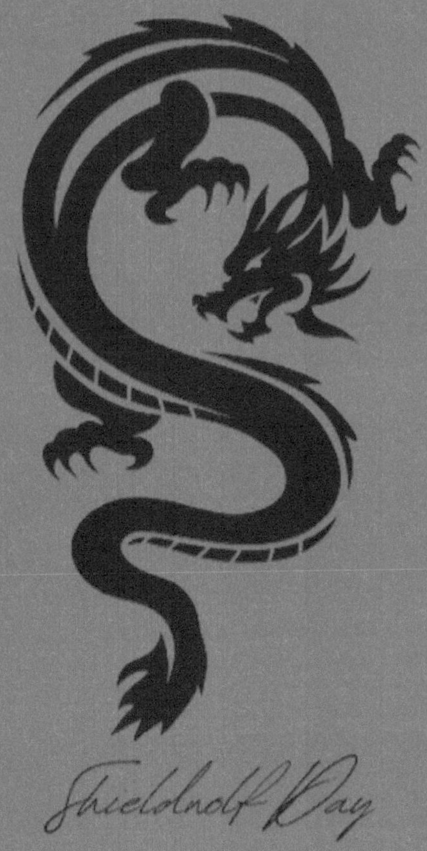

Shieldnolf Day

Becoming the Dragon

The Beginners Guide to Quick Fitness

Shieldwolf Day

Contents

Title Page
A Quick Introduction 1
Meditation 3
Preparing for Your Home Workouts 7
Warm-Up and Cool-Down 10
Individual Muscle Control 14
Becoming the Dragon 17
Bodyweight Exercises for Full-Body Fitness 20
Using Minimal Equipment for Maximum Impact 25
Structuring a ~30-Minute Workout Routine 29
Staying Motivated and Making Exercise a Habit 34
Adapting Your Workouts as You Progress 41
Overcoming Common Challenges and Staying Consistent 45
Nutrition Basics for Beginners 49
Resources and Tools for Success 53
Final Thoughts 56
Glossary of Terms 58

A Quick Introduction

Welcome to the first step of your fitness journey! This book is designed for anyone who is short on time but still wants to stay active and healthy. Whether you're a busy parent, juggling a full schedule, or just someone looking to fit in some quick movement to recenter yourself, this guide has you covered. You don't need a gym membership or fancy equipment- just your body, a little space, an open mind, and a little time.

The workouts in this book are for beginners, but even if you are getting back into fitness after a break, you will find them effective and easy to follow. These exercises focus on bodyweight movements that can be done anywhere, but there will also be sections that gloss over a few simple tools, like resistance bands and dumbbells, that you may want to get as you progress in your fitness journey.

The main thing I want to introduce you to is a technique I call *Becoming the Dragon*- hence the title of this book. We will be using meditation to help us achieve this state, and as I believe meditation is so important to overall health; I will cover that first.

But before that...

Why Work Out at Home?

Working out at home is all about convenience. No more commuting to an overcrowded gym or trying to squeeze a session into a packed schedule. You have the flexibility to work out on your own time, whenever you want to or need too. Plus, there's no need for bulky, expensive equipment- you can achieve great results using just your body or, if you choose to, minimal, affordable gear.

What Can You Expect?

In this book, you will find quick, efficient workouts that take minutes and can be done in between some of the tasks of your busy day. Whether you're looking to boost your energy or improve your strength, these routines are designed to fit into your life without overwhelming it. You'll find workouts that target all muscle groups to meditation to my own personal fitness technique, that if you master, you will never need anything else.

Now that we have covered that...

Let's Get Started!

Remember, fitness is about progress, not perfection. The key to success is showing up and putting in the time. Every workout counts, no matter how small. The best workout is the one you do. Let's make this fun, rewarding, and a part of your daily routine!

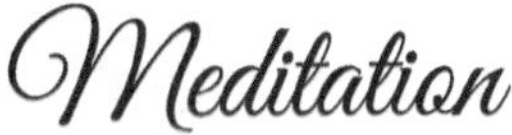

For Mind and Body Balance

Why Meditation?

Meditation isn't just for mental relaxation; it has a range of benefits that directly support physical fitness, such as reducing stress, improving sleep, and enhancing mental focus. By practicing meditation, you can boost your energy levels, increase motivation, and improve recovery time, helping you stay consistent with your fitness routine.

Let's dig a little deeper into those concepts.

Benefits of Meditation for Fitness

- **Reduced Stress and Anxiety:** Physical tension can be a byproduct of stress. Meditation helps calm the mind, releasing stress and improving physical relaxation.
- **Better Sleep:** Quality sleep is crucial for muscle recovery and energy levels. Meditation can promote better sleep (especially if done before bed) by relaxing the body and mind. Body Scan Meditation can help you drift to sleep.
- **Enhanced Focus:** Regular meditation helps improve concentration, making it easier to stay on track with workout routines and goals. Breathing Exercises can help you focus during stressful or chaotic moments throughout your day.
- **Increased Body Awareness:** Meditation cultivates mindfulness, which can help you pay more attention to form and movement, reducing the risk of injury. This is the

most important aspect for the technique I call Becoming the Dragon.

Getting Started with Meditation

You don't need much time or experience to start meditating. Keep in mind that everyone is different and that if a certain technique doesn't appeal or work for you, it's okay to try something new. It's important to not give up. Anyone can meditate, as long as you're open to the idea. Here are some simple methods to begin with:

- **Breathing Exercises:** Find a quiet space, close your eyes, and focus on your breath. Take a deep breath, hold it for a few seconds, then exhale slowly. Try this for five minutes, extend the time as needed.
- **Body Scan Meditation:** Starting at your feet, mentally "scan" each area of your body, consciously relaxing it as you go. This technique is great for after workouts to release any lingering tension.
- **Mindful Movement:** Integrate mindfulness with movement. Practice focusing on the way your body feels during exercises, noticing how each muscle works. This can improve form and enhance results.

Quick Guide Meditation Routines

Try this five minute meditation to unwind or prepare for a workout:

1. **Sit Comfortably:** Find a seated position, close your eyes, and relax your shoulders.
2. **Breathe Deeply:** Take a slow, deep breath in through your nose, hold, and the exhale through your mouth.
3. **Focus on Your Breathing:** Count your breaths up to 10. Note the sensation of each breath.
4. **Observe Without Judgment:** If your mind wanders,

gently bring it back to that sensation of breathing without frustration.

5. **End Slowly:** Open your eyes, take one final deep breath, and continue your day with renewed focus.

Second-

Try this visualization meditation if you find it hard to quiet your mind.

1. **Find a Comfortable, Quiet place:** Remain standing, close your eyes and relax your muscles.
2. **Breathe Deeply:** Take a slow, deep breath, hold for a half second then exhale.
3. **Visualize:** Observe the darkness of your closed eyes, now picture yourself standing amongst it.
4. **Imagine:** This part can be personalized, but for now, picture yourself as a tree. Your roots stretch deep into the earth. You draw in positive energy from the ground that helps you grow. You can visualize this as golden energy flowing into your feet then throughout your entire body.
5. **Finalization:** Stretch your arms and hands out, picturing your arms and fingers as branches reaching for the sunlight as you exhale the negative energies and thoughts that would stunt your growth.
6. **End Slowly:** Keep your eyes closed as you extend your senses. Attempt to feel the energies of everything around as you take a deep breath. Open your eyes as you exhale the last of the negative energies.

Lastly-

The meditation I personally use most often.

1. **Find a Comfortable Spot:** Find a quiet spot, if you need it. Put yourself in a relaxed position, standing or sitting.

2. **Focus:** Close your eyes and take a deep breath, focus on the stillness of the darkness before you.
3. **Visualize:** Picture a black hole in that darkness. Its pull is strong but so are you and you have no need to fear it.
4. **Imagine:** All of your negative thoughts, memories, regrets, and fears are being pulled away from you. The black hole greedily swallows them.
5. **Finalization:** Now that you're free from that weight, your body feels light. The darkness around you opens up revealing the stars of endless space. You are free to extend your senses out into that space or to turn them inward.
6. **End Slowly:** Keep your senses extended, inward or outward, as you open your eyes. Take a few deep, patient breaths as you let your senses relax.

There's as many ways to meditate as there are people. If you find yourself struggling, try creating your own methods. You can also tailor someone else's technique to you or listen to a guided meditation.

I have personally thought about making a series of guided meditations on YouTube. If that would appeal to you, feel free to let me know in your review of this book.

Now that we have covered, let's move on to the more physical side of working out.

Preparing for Your Home Workouts

Before jumping into your first workout, it's important to set up your space and have everything you need ready to go. Don't worry- getting prepared is simple, and you don't need a dedicated gym space to make this work. Here are a few tips to help you get started:

1. **Find Your Workout Space**

You don't need a lot of room to exercise- just enough to comfortably move around without bumping into furniture. Clear a small area where you can stretch your arms and legs without obstruction. A living room, bedroom, or even a hallway can work perfectly. If you have a yoga mat, use it for extra comfort on hard floors.

2. **Minimal Equipment Needed (Optional)**

The majority of exercises in this book require no equipment at all, but having a few affordable items can add variety and challenge to your routine. Here's what you might want to consider:

Resistance Bands: Lightweight and affordable, these are great for adding resistance to bodyweight exercises, helping you build strength and endurance without heavy weights.
Dumbbells: If you're looking to build strength, a pair of light dumbbells (5-10lbs) can be a great addition for exercises like squats or lunges.
Chair or Sturdy Surface: Many exercises, like step-ups or tricep dips, can be done using a chair or bench you already have at home.
Towel or Mat: A yoga mat or towel can make floor exercises more comfortable, especially for things like planks or sit-ups.

3. Wear Comfortable Clothing

One of the perks of working out at home is that there's no dress code! You don't need fancy workout gear- just wear something comfortable that allows you to move freely. Sneakers are ideal for most workouts, but if you're doing yoga or pilates-based movements, barefoot or socks with grip might feel better.

4. Hydration and Safety

Even though you're at home, staying hydrated is just as important as if you were in the gym. Keep a bottle of water nearby and take sips throughout your workout.

Safety Tips for Beginners:

- **Listen to Your Body:** Pay attention to how you feel during each exercise. If something doesn't feel right or causes pain, stop immediately. It's better to modify an exercise or skip it than to risk injury.
- **Focus on Form:** Quality over quantity is key. It's more beneficial to perform fewer reps with proper form than to do many reps incorrectly. Take your time to learn the movements correctly.
- **Take Breaks:** Don't hesitate to take breaks as needed, especially if you're feeling fatigued. This helps prevent injury and ensures you're up and able for your next workout.

5. Warm-Up and Cool-Down

Every workout should start with a short warm-up and end with a cool-down to keep your muscles healthy and prevent injury. We will cover some simple routines for both in the next section.

6. Set Yourself Up for Success

Creating a consistent workout routine is key to making fitness a lasting part of your life. Consider scheduling your workouts at times that fit best with your day, whether it's in the morning before your responsibilities kick in, during your lunch break, or in the evening after dinner. Treat these workout times as appointments that you can't miss.

Warm-Up and Cool-Down

Every workout- whether it's short or long- should start with a proper warm-up and end with a cool-down. These simple routines are often overlooked but are crucial for preventing injury, improving performance, and helping your body recover. Think of your warm-up as preparing your body for movement, and the cool-down as helping it ease back into rest.

Warm-Up Routine

A good warm-up gets your blood flowing, increases your heart rate, and loosens up your muscles, making them more flexible and ready for movement. Here's a quick five-minute warm-up you can do before any workout:

- **March in Place (~one minute):**
  Start by standing tall with your feet hip-width apart. Begin to march in place, lifting your knees as high as you comfortably can with each step. Engage your core by flexing your abs slightly and keep your chest lifted. As you march, swing your arms forward and backwards naturally to activate your upper body. This movement gently elevates your heart rate and starts warming up your legs, core, and shoulders.

- **Arm Circles (~30 seconds each direction):**
  Stand with your feet shoulder-width apart and extend your arms out to the sides at shoulder height, keeping them straight but relaxed. Begin to circle your arms forward, making small circles at first, then gradually making them larger. After 30 seconds, reverse the direction of the circles, starting big and then shrinking them. This exercise warms

up the shoulders and loosens the muscles around your upper back and chest, preparing you for upper-body exercises.

- **Leg Swings (~30 seconds per leg):**
  Stand next to a wall or sturdy surface for balance. Shift your weight onto one leg and begin to swing the other leg forward and backward in a controlled manner. As you swing, make sure to keep your hips facing forward and avoid overextending. This dynamic stretch helps open up your hip flexors and hamstrings, which are key for lower body exercises. After 30 seconds, switch legs and repeat.

- **Torso Twists (~ 1 minute):**
  Stand with your feet slightly wider than shoulder-width apart, and place your hands at your sides or gently on your hips. Slowly twist your torso from left to right, allowing your arms to swing freely with the movement. Engage your core and keep your knees slightly bent. This exercise increases mobility in your spine and warms up your oblique muscles, which are important for stabilizing the body during many movements.

- **Bodyweight Squats (~1 minute):**
  Stand with your feet shoulder-width apart, toes pointing slightly outward. Push your hips back as if you're sitting down into a chair, keeping your chest up and back straight. Lower yourself until your thighs are parallel to the ground, then push through your heels to stand back up. Focus on keeping your knees aligned with your toes and avoid letting them cave inward. Bodyweight squats are great for warming up your quads, hamstrings, glutes, and core.

Cool-Down Routine

After your workout, it's important to bring your heart rate down and stretch out your muscles. Cooling down helps prevent stiffness and improve flexibility. Here's a quick five minute cool-down routine:

- **Slow Walking or Marching (~1 minute):**
After your workout, take a minute to slowly walk around or march in place. Keep your movements gentle and controlled, allowing your heart rate to gradually decrease. This helps prevent dizziness and gives your body time to transition from high-intensity exercise to rest.

- **Quad Stretch (~30 seconds per leg):**
Stand on one leg and grab the ankle of your opposite leg, pulling your heel toward your glutes. Keep your knees close together and push your hips slightly forward to deepen the stretch. Hold onto a wall or chair for balance if needed. You should feel a stretch along the front of your thigh (quadriceps). After 30 seconds, switch legs. This stretch helps relax the muscles that worked hard during exercises like squats or lunges.

- **Hamstring Stretch (~1 minute):**
Sit on the floor with one leg extended in front of you and the other bent, with the sole of your foot resting against the inside of your thigh. Slowly reach toward your toes on the extended leg, keeping your back straight and hinging from your hips. You should feel a stretch along the back of your thigh (hamstrings). Hold for 30 seconds, then switch sides. This stretch helps release tension in the hamstrings, which are often tight after leg exercises.

- **Shoulder Stretch (~30 seconds per arm):**
Extend one arm across your chest at shoulder height. Use your opposite hand to gently pull the arm closer to your chest, feeling the stretch along the back of your shoulder and upper back. Hold for 30 seconds, then switch arms. This stretch is particularly beneficial after any upper-body exercises like push-ups or planks, helping to release tightness in the shoulders and upper back.

- **Child's Pose (~1 minute):**

Kneel on the floor with your knees spread wide, big toes touching behind you. Sit back onto your heels and reach your arms forward, lowering your chest toward the ground. Allow your forehead to rest on the floor and relax into the stretch. This pose stretches your lower back, shoulders, and hips, making it a perfect way to wind down after a workout.

Individual Muscle Control

Now that we've covered warm-up's and cool-down's, let's move on to one of the core components for the technique I am most excited to teach you, "Becoming the Dragon".

What Is Individual Muscle Control?

Individual muscle control, or "muscle activation", is the practice of isolating and engaging specific muscles during exercise. Instead of just performing movements, you learn to focus on each muscle being used, which leads to better form, increased strength, and reduced risk of injury.

Benefits of Developing Muscle Control

- **Improved Strength Gains:** Targeting specific muscles more accurately can improve muscle activation, leading to greater gains and better muscle tone.
- **Better Exercise Form:** Focusing on muscle control can ensure that each movement is performed safely and effectively, reducing strain on joints.
- **Enhanced Mind-Muscle Control:** A stronger mind-muscle connection allows for better focus, which can improve workout intensity and overall results.

How to Practice Muscle Control

Here are a few exercises to help you develop control over individual muscles:

Mind-Muscle Warm-Up: Start each workout by warming up with light movements (like bodyweight squats or arm circles) while paying attention to the muscle being engaged. This primes your mind-muscle connection for the workout.

Isometric Holds: Holding a position engages muscles deeply. Try holding a plank or a squat position for 15 to 30 seconds, focusing on the specific muscles working to maintain the hold.

Slow, Controlled Movements: Perform exercises slowly to increase the time under tension. For example, in a push-up, take 3 seconds to lower down and 3 seconds to push back up, focusing on your chest, shoulders, and arms.

Plank (Core, Shoulders)

Focus on tightening your abs and glutes.
Press your hands into the ground, feeling your shoulders engage.
Keep your body in a straight line, resist any sagging.

Squats (Glutes, Hamstrings, Quadriceps)

Engage your glutes and quadriceps as you lower.
Press through your heels as you stand, focusing on activating your glutes.
Visualize your glutes and quads working together to lift you.

Bicep Curls (Biceps)

Move slowly, squeezing your biceps at the top of the curl.
Focus on lowering the weight with control, resisting gravity.

Bridge (Glutes, Hamstrings)

As you lift your hips, engage your glutes.
Focus on the hamstrings and glutes working together to hold the position.
Avoid letting your lower back do the work by tightening your abs.

Practice Tips for Muscle Control

- **Visualize Each Muscle Group:** Before starting a movement, visualize the muscle you're about to work. This mental focus strengthens the connections between your mind and body.

- **Contract and Release:** Practice tightening and relaxing muscles, even outside of workouts. This helps you identify specific muscles and learn how to engage them consciously.
- **Focus on Form Over Speed:** Slow down your movements during workouts. This allows you to feel each muscle's activation and helps build control.

Putting it All Together

Improving individual muscle control takes practice, but it can make a big difference in how effective and safe your workouts are. With consistency, you'll build strength and improve your overall body awareness, making each exercise more efficient and rewarding.

Becoming the Dragon

Now that we've covered the basics, let's get into the technique itself. As you might have guessed, Becoming the Dragon is a blend of individual muscle control, meditation, and movement. Don't worry if these aspects didn't stick with you or didn't appeal to you; I also included more foundational exercises in the rest of this guidebook.

Why call it Becoming the Dragon? Because this is about transformation, both physically and mentally. Remember, this is your journey, and Becoming the Dragon is all about making the technique your own. As you practice, it will evolve into something uniquely yours.

Getting started may take about 10 minutes, but as you gain confidence and familiarity, the process will become quicker and more natural.

Beginning the Transformation

Start with a brief meditation. Close your eyes while you mentally "scan" your body. Start with your feet, moving slowly upward , focusing on each muscle group. If it helps, give each muscle a gentle flex as you pass over it.

Keep your eyes closed as you finish. Visualize a dragon or whichever symbol of power and strength resonates with you.

You are going to become this paragon of strength.

Picture the dragon's muscles rippling under its skin, see them popping up through its scales. Imagine its strength flowing through you. Flex your muscles with the dragon. It is you.

Awakening the Dragon

Open your eyes, keeping the image of the dragon firmly in your mind. Begin stretching, but not just any stretch- stretch as though you are the dragon. Feel your muscles ripple with strength. Visualize yourself becoming more agile, powerful, and focused with every one of your warm-ups. This is your time to channel the presence and energy of the dragon.

Move Like the Dragon

Transition into your bodyweight exercises while maintaining your focus on the dragon. Move deliberately and with control. Start slowly, paying attention to each movement and how your muscles engage. This isn't a race- it's a process. With time, you'll grow into the strength and fluidity of the dragon.

As you master this technique, the more natural it will become to you. You will be able to integrate it seamlessly into your workouts. Eventually, you will be able to flex your muscles at any time for a workout. You will be able to workout without any exercises at all or by doing simple movements.

Tips:

- **Focus on Growth:** If you're struggling to flex specific muscles, don't worry. It might simply mean you need to build more strength in that area first. Try doing some of the exercises listed in the next section to build a base for you to work from.
- **Don't Stress:** If you find you're having a hard time with the technique, try normal exercises and try again a different day. It's okay to not do the technique everyday or to come back to it when you feel more open to it.
- **Personalize:** This technique works best when it feels meaningful to you. Maybe a dragon doesn't resonate, but a tiger, a grizzly bear, or even a strong, enduring oak tree does. The choice is yours. Whatever you choose, make it mean

something to you, as long as you have a connection the more likely you are to see results.
- **Cool-Down:** Don't forget to do a cool-down!

For me, this practice has evolved into something I can do anytime, anywhere. On a rest day, I might flow through slow Tai Chi movements while flexing individual muscles. On a work out day, I'll shadow box with specific muscles engaged. The beauty of Becoming the Dragon is that it's yours to shape and grow.

Bodyweight Exercises for Full-Body Fitness

Bodyweight exercises are incredibly effective because they use your own body as resistance. They not only help build strength but also improve balance, flexibility, and endurance. The best part? No equipment is needed! Below are some foundational exercises that target major muscle groups, making them perfect for a complete workout at home.

Push-Ups

Target Areas: Chest, shoulders, triceps, and core

How to Do It:
Start in a high plank position with your hands placed slightly wider than shoulder-width apart, fingers pointing forward. Keep your body in a straight line from head to heels, engaging your core and squeezing your glutes. Lower your body toward the floor by bending your elbows, keeping them at a 45-degree angle to your torso.

Squats

Target Areas: Quads, glutes, hamstrings, and core

How to Do It:
Stand with your feet shoulder-width apart and toes slightly pointing out. Lower your body by bending your knees and

pushing your hips back, as if sitting in an invisible chair. Keep your chest lifted and your back straight, making sure your knees track over your toes. Lower down until your thighs are parallel to the floor (or as low as you can go), then push through your heels to return to standing.

Tip: Engage your core throughout the movement to maintain stability and avoid straining your lower back.

Plank

Target Areas: Core, shoulder, and glutes

How to Do It:

Start by lying face down on the floor, then come up onto your forearms and toes, elbows directly under your shoulders. Keep your body in a straight line from your head to your heels, with your core fully engaged. Hold this position without letting your hips drop or rise too high.

Goal: Aim to hold the plank for 20-30 seconds to start and gradually increase your time as you get stronger.

Lunges

Target Areas: Quads, glutes, hamstrings, and calves

How to Do It:

Stand tall with your feet together and take a big step forward with one leg. Lower your body until your front knee is bent at 90 degrees and your back knee is just above the floor. Push through your front heel to return to the starting position, then switch legs.

Tip: Keep your torso upright and avoid leaning forward you can also add a slight pause at the bottom of the movement to engage your muscles more.

Glute Bridges

Target Areas: Glutes, hamstrings, and lower back

How to Do It:

Lie on your back with your knees bent and feet flat on the floor, hip-width apart. Press your heels into the floor and lift your hips toward the ceiling, squeezing your glutes at the top. Hold for a second at the top, then slowly lower hips back down to the floor. That's one rep.

Tip: To increase difficulty, try doing single-leg glute bridges by extending one leg in the air while lifting your hips.

Superman

Target Areas: Glutes, hamstrings, and lower back

How to Do It:

Lie face down on the floor with your arms extended straight in front of you and your legs extended behind. Simultaneously lift your arms, chest, and legs off the floor, engaging your glutes and lower back. Hold for 1-2 seconds at the top, then lower back down. This movement helps strengthen your back muscles, which are often overlooked.

Mountain Climbers

Target Areas: Core, shoulders, and legs

How to Do It:

Start in a high plank position with your hands under your shoulders and your body in a straight line. Drive one knee toward your chest, then quickly switch legs, bringing the opposite knee forward while pushing the other leg back. Continue alternating legs in a running motion, keeping your core tight and hips low.

Tip: Maintain a controlled pace at first, then speed up as you get more comfortable. This exercise also adds a cardio element to your routine.

Tricep Dips

Target Areas: Triceps, shoulders, and chest

How to Do It:
Sit on the edge of a sturdy chair or low bench with your hands gripping the edge, fingers facing forward. Slide your hips off the chair and lower your body by bending your elbows until your upper arms are parallel to the floor. Push back up to the starting position by straightening your arms.

Tip: Keep your elbows tucked in close to your body to target the triceps effectively. To make it more challenging, straighten your legs out in front of you.

Bicycle Crunches

Target Areas: Abs and obliques

How to Do It:

Lie on your back with your knees bent and hands behind your head. Lift your shoulder blades off the floor and bring one knee toward your chest while simultaneously twisting your torso to bring the opposite elbow toward the knee. Switch sides, extending the other leg and bringing the opposite elbow to the other knee.

Tip: Focus on controlled movements and engage your core throughout the exercise. Avoid pulling on your neck to prevent strain.

Burpees

Target Areas: Full body (legs, arms, chest, and core)

How to Do It:
Stand with your feet shoulder-width apart. Lower your body into a squat and place your hands on the floor in front of you. Jump your feet back into a plank position, then lower your chest to the floor for a push-up. Push back up and jump your feet forward, then explode upward in a jump, reaching your arms overhead.

Tip: If you're just starting out, you can skip the push-up or the jump until you build strength.

Using Minimal Equipment for Maximum Impact

While bodyweight exercises are highly effective, adding a few affordable pieces of equipment can take your workouts to the next level. You don't need a fully stocked gym to see results- just a few key items that are inexpensive, portable, and easy to use at home.

Resistance Bands

Why Use Them:
Resistance bands are versatile, affordable, and take up almost no space. They come in different levels of resistance, making them great for beginners and advanced users alike. Resistance bands are perfect for adding extra challenge to your bodyweight exercises, improving strength, and enhancing muscle tone.

How to Use Them:

- **Squats with Resistance Bands:** Place a resistance band just above your knees. Perform a standard squat, but as you lower, push your knees outward against the resistance band. This helps activate your glutes and outer thighs.

- **Banded Glute Bridges:** Wrap the band above your knees and lie on your back for a glute bridge. The added resistance makes your glutes work harder as you lift your hips.

- **Bicep Curls:** Stand in the middle of a resistance band with both feet. Hold the ends in your hands and curl your arms up toward your shoulders. This simple move strengthens your arms without the need for dumbbells.

Dumbbells

Why Use Them:
Dumbbells are a great addition to your home workout setup. They come in various weights, allowing you to gradually increase resistance as you get stronger. Dumbbells are excellent for targeting specific muscles and can be used for a wide variety of exercises.

How to Use Them:

- **Dumbbell Deadlifts:** Hold a dumbbell in each hand, standing with your feet hip-width apart. Hinge at the hips, lowering the dumbbells toward the floor while keeping your back straight. This targets your hamstrings and glutes.
- **Dumbbell Shoulder Press:** Hold a dumbbell in each hand at shoulder height, palms facing forward. Press the dumbbells overhead, fully extending your arms, and then lower them back down. This works your shoulders and upper arms.
- **Goblet Squats:** Hold a single dumbbell vertically in front of your chest with both hands. Perform a squat, keeping the dumbbell close to your body. This variation adds extra resistance to your lower-body workout.

Jump Rope

Why Use It:
Jump ropes are one of the best cardio tools out there. They're cheap, portable, and deliver an incredible full-body workout. Jumping rope improves your cardiovascular fitness, coordination, and balance, all while burning calories.

How to Use It:
Before starting any jump rope exercises, make sure you have ample space. You may want to consider doing these exercises outside.

- **Basic Jumping:** Start with both feet together, holding the handles of the rope at your sides. Rotate your wrists to swing the rope overhead and jump as it passes under your feet. Keep your jumps small and light to conserve energy.

- **Alternate-Foot Jumps:** Instead of jumping with both feet, alternate between landing on your left and right foot, mimicking a running motion. This variation boosts agility and endurance.

Stability Ball

Why Use It:
A stability ball (also called a Swiss ball) is great for improving balance, core strength, and flexibility. It adds an element of instability to your exercises, forcing your muscles to work harder to maintain control.

How to Use It:

- **Ball Rollouts:** Kneel on the floor with your forearms resting on the stability ball. Slowly roll the ball forward, extending your body into a plank position, then roll it back. This exercise engages your core and improves balance.
- **Stability Ball Planks:** Place your forearms on the stability ball while in a plank position. The instability of the ball increases the challenge, engaging your core and shoulders even more.
- **Wall Squats with Stability Ball:** Place the ball between your lower back and a wall. Lean against the ball and squat down, using the ball to support your movement. This targets your legs and improves lower body control.

Kettlebells

Why Use Them:
Kettlebells are incredibly versatile and provide a combination of strength training and cardiovascular conditioning. Their unique shape allows for swinging movements that activate multiple muscle groups at once, making them great for functional fitness.

How to Use Them:

- **Kettlebell Swings:** Hold a kettlebell with both hands in front of your hips. Swing it backward between your legs, then drive your hips forward to swing it up to chest level. This powerful movement targets your glutes, hamstrings, and core while providing a cardio boost.
- **Kettle Deadlifts:** Similar to dumbbell deadlifts, but with the kettlebell in both hands between your legs, then drive your hips forward to swing it up to chest level. This powerful movement targets your glutes, hamstrings, and core while providing a cardio boost.
- **Goblet Squat:** Hold the kettlebell close to your chest and perform a squat. The weight of the kettlebell adds resistance and helps improve your squatting form.

Structuring a ~30-Minute Workout Routine

Time is precious, especially for beginners, busy parents, and those juggling hectic schedules. But even with just 30 minutes a day, you can get an effective workout that targets your whole body, builds strength, and boosts fitness. Here's how to structure your quick, efficient workouts:

Warm-Up (5 minutes)

A proper warm-up prepares your body exercise, increases blood flow to your muscles, and helps prevent injury. The goal is to gradually increase your heart rate and loosen up your muscles.

Sample Warm-Up Routine:

- **Jumping Jacks (1 minute):** Start with a full-body movement to elevate your heart rate.
- **Arm Circles (30 seconds forward, 30 seconds backward):** Stand with arms outstretched and move them in small circles to loosen your shoulders.
- **Leg Swings (1 minute):** Stand on one leg and swing the other forward and backward, then switch sides.
- **Bodyweight Squats (1 minute):** Perform slow, controlled squats to warm up your legs and glutes.
- **High Knees (1 minute):** March in place, lifting your knees toward your chest, to activate your hip flexors and engage your core.

Circuit Training (20 minutes)

Circuit training is an efficient way to combine strength and cardio into one workout. Perform each exercise for 40 seconds, then rest for 20 seconds before moving to the next one. After completing the circuit, rest for 1-2 minutes and repeat it 2-3 times, depending on your fitness level.

Sample Circuit:[1]

- **Push-Ups**- 40 seconds of work
- **Squats**- 40 seconds of work
- **Plank**- 40 seconds of holding
- **Lunges**- 40 seconds of alternating legs
- **Glute Bridges**- 40 seconds of work
- **Mountain Climbers**- 40 seconds of work

Tips for Circuit Training:

- **Go at your own pace.** The goal is to maintain good form, not rush through the exercises. As you get stronger, you can increase your speed and intensity.
- **Modify exercises as needed.** If you're struggling with any movement, try a modified version. For example, use knee push-ups if regular push-ups are too tough.
- **Rest between circuits.** Don't skip the rest periods- these short breaks help you maintain stamina for the full workout.

Cool-Down (5 Minutes)

Cooling down is just as important as warming up. It helps reduce muscle stiffness, improves flexibility, and allows your heart rate to gradually return to normal.

Sample Cool-Down Routine:

- **Forward Fold Stretch (1 minute):** Stand tall, bend at the hips, and reach for your toes. Let your upper body hang, stretching your hamstrings and lower back.

- **Quad Stretch (30 seconds each leg):** Stand on one leg and pull your opposite foot toward your glutes, stretching the front of your thigh.
- **Cat-Cow Stretch (1 minute):** Start on your hands and knees. Arch your back (cat pose), then dip it toward the floor as you look up (cow pose). This stretches your spine and loosens your lower back.
- **Child's Pose (1 minute):** Kneel on the floor, sit back on your heels, and stretch your arms forward, letting your chest drop toward the floor. This gentle stretch relaxes your body.

Sample Weekly Workout Plans

Creating a structured workout plan can make it easier to stay consistent and ensure a balanced approach to fitness. Below are three sample workout plans tailored for different fitness levels: beginner, intermediate, and advanced. Each plan focuses on a mix of bodyweight exercises and cheap equipment to keep things accessible.

Beginner Workout Plan

Goal: Establish a routine and build foundational strength.

Weekly Schedule:

- **Monday:** Full-Body Bodyweight Workout (30 minutes)
- **Tuesday:** Active Recovery (e.g., walking or light stretching)
- **Wednesday:** Core Workout (30 minutes)
- **Thursday:** Cardio (e.g., jogging in place or brisk walking for 30 minutes)
- **Friday:** Full-Body Workout with Dumbbells (30 minutes)
- **Saturday:** Active Recovery (yoga or light stretching)
- **Sunday:** Rest Day

Intermediate Workout Plan

Goal: Increase strength and endurance with added resistance.

Weekly Schedule:

- **Monday:** Full-Body Resistance Workout (30 minutes with dumbbells and resistance bands)
- **Tuesday:** HIIT (30 minutes, alternating between high-intensity exercises and rest)
- **Wednesday:** Core and Flexibility (30 minutes of core work followed by yoga)
- **Thursday:** Cardio (30 minutes of cycling or brisk walking)
- **Friday:** Lower Body Focus (30 minutes of squats, lunges, and resistance bands)
- **Saturday:** Active Recovery (light activities or leisure sports)
- **Sunday:** Rest Day

Advanced Workout Plan

Goal: Challenge strength and endurance with a mix of workouts.

Weekly Schedule:

- **Monday:** Upper Body Strength and Core (30 minutes of bodyweight and dumbbell exercises)
- **Tuesday:** HIIT/Cardio Blast (30 minutes of varied cardio exercises)
- **Wednesday:** Lower Body Strength and Flexibility (30 minutes of advanced bodyweight exercises)
- **Thursday:** Full-Body Circuit (30 minutes of alternating bodyweight and resistance exercises)
- **Friday:** Cardio Endurance (45 minutes of running, cycling, or swimming)
- **Saturday:** Active Recovery (yoga or light stretching)
- **Sunday:** Rest Day

Common Mistakes to Avoid

Being aware of common mistakes can help beginners stay on track and avoid setbacks. Here are some pitfalls to watch out for:

- **Skipping Warm-Ups and Cool Downs:** Neglecting these crucial parts of your workout can lead to injuries and hinder recovery. Always take a few minutes to warm up your muscles and cool down afterward.
- **Overtraining:** Pushing yourself too hard without adequate rest can lead to burnout and injuries. Remember that recovery is as important as training—incorporate rest days into your routine.
- **Focusing Solely on One Type of Exercise:** Doing only cardio or strength training can create imbalances. Aim for a well-rounded routine that includes various exercises for overall fitness.
- **Setting Unrealistic Goals:** While ambition is great, setting goals that are too lofty can lead to disappointment. Start with smaller, achievable goals, and gradually progress as you build confidence and fitness.
- **Ignoring Nutrition:** Exercise alone won't yield desired results if nutrition isn't addressed. Focus on a balanced diet that supports your fitness goals, including adequate protein, healthy fats, and carbohydrates.

Staying Motivated and Making Exercise a Habit

Starting a fitness journey is exciting, but staying consistent can be the biggest challenge. Motivation may come and go, but turning exercise into a habit is key to long-term success. Here are some tips to help you stay on track and make fitness a permanent part of your routine.

Set Realistic Goals

Setting achievable goals gives you something to work toward and keeps you motivated. Start with small, specific targets and build up from there. Goals give you direction and purpose, but if they are too ambitious, they can lead to frustration and a lack of motivation.

How to set Goals

- **S.M.A.R.T Goals:** Make your goals Specific, Measurable, Achievable, Relevant, and Time-bound. For example, instead of saying, "I want to get fit," set a goal like "I will complete at least three 30-minute workouts each week for the next month."
- **Break it down:** Divide larger goals into smaller, more manageable milestones.

Examples of Realistic Goals:

- Complete three workouts a week for the next month.
- Hold a plank for 30 seconds without dropping.

- Increase the number of push-ups you can do by two every week.

By focusing on small milestones, you'll see progress faster, which helps maintain your motivation. As you reach your goals, set new ones to keep challenging yourself.

<u>**Create a Schedule**</u>

One of the biggest barriers to regular exercise is lack of time. By Scheduling your workouts like appointments, you're more likely to stick to them. Look at your daily routine and find a 30-minute window that works for you- whether it's early in the morning, during lunch breaks, or after the kids go to bed. Years ago, when I was cooking dinner was the perfect time for me to nail out a workout in between cooking.

Tips for Scheduling:

- Pick consistent workout days and times to make it part of your routine. This will make it a habit. Your body will start to expect it, making it easier to stick to your plan.
- Treat your workout as a non-negotiable part of your day. Just like you would for work or other commitments, set aside specific time blocks for your workout.
- If something comes up, have a backup plan (like a shorter 15-minute workout or a backup time). Be flexible, life can be unpredictable. If you miss a workout, don't be too hard on yourself- just reschedule it to a different day.

<u>**Make it Fun**</u>

Exercise doesn't have to feel like a chore. Find ways to make your workouts enjoyable, whether it's by mixing up your routine, playing your favorite music, or turning it into a game.

Ideas for Adding Fun to Your Workouts:

- **Listen to music or a podcast:** A great playlist or podcast can make the time fly by.

- **Try new exercises:** Don't be afraid to experiment with different types of workouts to keep things interesting. Trying new exercises or workout formats can keep things exciting and fun.
- **Workout with a friend:** Having a workout buddy adds a social element and you can motivate each other. Invite friends or family to join you or you can join a local fitness group.

Fun Fitness Challenges

Engaging in fitness challenges can add excitement to your routine and foster a sense of community. Here are a few fun challenges you can try:

- **30-Day Squat Challenge:** Start with a manageable number of squats (e.g., 10) and increase the count every few days. By the end of the month, you'll be surprised at how many you can do!
- **Plank Challenge:** Aim to hold a plank for increasing durations each day. Start with 20 seconds and gradually increase to a minute or more.
- **Step Challenge:** Use a pedometer or fitness tracker to set a daily step goal. Encourage friends or family to join in and compete for the most steps each week.
- **Workout Bingo:** Create a bingo card filled with various exercises (e.g., push-ups, burpees, jumping jacks). Mark off squares as you complete each exercise, aiming to get a bingo within a month.

Track Your Progress

Keeping track of your workouts helps you see how far you've come. It's easy to overlook the improvements you're making, so having a visual reminder of your progress can be a huge motivator.

Ways to Track Progress:

- **Use a journal:** Write down the exercises you did, how many reps, and how you felt after each session.
- **Take progress photos:** sometimes, physical changes aren't immediately noticeable, but photos can show the subtle differences over time.
- **Track performance:** Record how long you held a plank, how many squats you completed, or the amount of weight you used. Seeing those numbers improve will inspire you to keep going.

Weekly Reflection Prompts

Incorporating reflection into your fitness journey can help reinforce positive habits. Here are some prompts to consider each week:

- **What were my biggest accomplishments this week?**
- **What challenges did I face, and how did I overcome them?**
- **How did I feel physically and mentally after my workouts?**
- **What exercise did I enjoy the most, and why?**
- **What goals do I want to set for next week?**

Stay Inspired

Finding sources of inspiration cna keep you motivated and help you overcome challenges as they present themselves.

Tips for staying inspired:

- **Follow fitness influencers:** Look for fitness bloggers, YouTube channels, or instagram accounts that resonate with you and provide motivation and workout ideas.
- **Join online communities:** Participate in forums or social media groups where you can share experiences, challenges, and successes with people on similar journeys.

- **Read success stories:** Inspirational stories of others who have achieved their fitness goals can remind you that progress is possible and motivate you to keep going.

Be Kind to Yourself

Life gets busy, and there will be days when you miss a workout, or don't feel like exercising. That's okay! The key is not to be too hard on yourself. Missing a day or two doesn't mean you've failed- it's just a part of the process.

Tips for Staying Kind to Yourself:

- **Practice self-compassion:** Accept that everyone has ups and downs. Be gentle with yourself when things don't go as planned.
- **Don't strive for perfection:** Focus on consistency, not perfection. A missed workout isn't the end of the world; just get back to it the next day.
- **Celebrate small victories:** Every time you show up for a workout, you're building the habit. Celebrate those small wins!
- **Listen to your body:** If you're feeling overly tired or sore, it's okay to take a rest day. Rest is, in part, progress.
- **Reflect on your journey:** Regularly remind yourself of why you started and how far you've come. This can help reignite your motivation.

Reward Yourself

Rewarding yourself for sticking to your routine can keep you motivated, especially when the going gets tough. Choose rewards that are meaningful and supportive of your fitness goals.

Reward Ideas:

- **New workout gear:** Treat yourself to a new pair of workout shoes or comfy activewear.
- **Non-food rewards:** Take time for a relaxing bath, watch your

favorite show, or enjoy some extra "me time".
- **Celebrate milestones:** When you hit a major goal (like completing your first month of consistent workouts), celebrate with a fun activity, like a day trip or trying a new class.

Focus on How You Feel

One of the best ways to stay motivated is by focusing on the benefits that exercise brings to your mental and physical health. While physical changes may take time, the immediate benefits, like reduced stress, better sleep, and more energy, are often felt after just a few workouts.

How Exercise Makes You Feel Better:

- **Boosts your mood:** Exercise releases endorphins, the body's natural feel-good chemicals.
- **Improves sleep quality:** Regular physical activity can help you fall asleep faster and improve the quality of your sleep.
- **Increases energy:** While it might seem counterintuitive, exercise can boost your energy levels, making it easier to tackle daily tasks.

Embrace Rest and Recovery

Remember that rest and recovery are just as important as exercise. Your body needs time to recover, repair, and grow stronger. Avoid burnout by incorporating rest days into your routine.

Tips for Rest and Recovery

- **Schedule rest days:** Plan regular rest days each week to allow your muscles to recover and prevent injury.
- **Listen to your body:** If you're feeling fatigued, sore, or unmotivated, take an extra rest day or opt for a lighter workout.
- **Recovery techniques:** Incorporate activities like stretching, foam rolling, or gentle yoga on rest days to aid recovery and

enhance flexibility.

Adapting Your Workouts as You Progress

As you get stronger and fitter, your body will adapt to the exercises, and what once felt challenging will start to feel easier. To keep improving and prevent plateaus, it's important to adjust your workouts to match your progress. Here's how to keep pushing your limits without overdoing it.

Focus on Form and Technique

Progress isn't just about lifting heavier or doing more reps- it's also about improving the quality of your movements. As you advance, pay extra attention to your form. Proper form helps you avoid injury and ensures you're engaging the correct muscles.

Tips for Improving Form:

Record yourself: Sometimes you don't realize your form is off until you see it. Recording a few of your movements can help you spot areas you need improvement in.
Slow down: Slowing down the movement (especially during exercises like push-ups, lunges, or squats) allows you to focus on your form and increase time under tension, which helps build muscle.
Engage your core: In most exercises, your core should be actively engaged to protect your spine and enhance stability.

Increase Repetitions and Sets

One of the simplest ways to progress is by increasing the number of repetitions (reps) or adding more sets of each exercise.

This gradual increase ensures that your muscles are continually challenged.

How to Progress:

- **Add reps:** If you're doing 10 push-ups, try adding 2-3 more each week. This small increase builds strength over time.
- **Add sets:** If you're used to doing 2 sets of an exercise increase it to 3 sets as you feel stronger.

Increase Intensity

Adding intensity can make your workouts more effective without needing extra time. This could mean reducing rest time between exercises, increasing the speed of each movement, or making the exercise more explosive.

How to Increase Intensity

- **Decrease rest:** Shorten rest periods between exercises (for example, from 40 seconds to 30 seconds).
- **Add speed:** For movements like squats, lunges, or burpees, increase the tempo to challenge your endurance and agility.
- **Explosive moves:** incorporate plyometrics, like jump squats or jump lunges, to increase intensity and engage more muscles.

Try Advanced Variations

Once the basic versions of exercises start to feel too easy, it's time to challenge yourself with more advanced variations. This ensures you continue building strength and endurance.

Advanced Exercise Variations:

- **Push-ups:** Move from knee push-ups to regular push-ups, and eventually to more advanced versions like decline push-ups or clap push-ups.
- **Squats:** Add a jump to turn your squats into squat jumps, or try single-leg pistol squats for a balance challenge.
- **Planks:** Try side planks or add movement, like alternating leg

raises, to increase difficulty.

Add Resistance

Introducing external resistance, such as resistance bands, dumbbells, or kettlebells, is a great way to keep progressing. This adds extra load, making your muscles work harder.

How to Add Resistance:

- **Use resistance bands:** As mentioned earlier[2], you can add bands to squats, lunges, and glute bridges for a greater challenge.
- **Increase weight:** If you've been using dumbbells, gradually increase the weight. For example, if you started with 5-pound dumbbells, move to 8 or 10 pounds when the lighter weights become easy.
- **Kettlebell exercises:** Adding kettlebells to your routine, especially for movements like kettlebell swings or goblet squats, can increase overall strength and power.

Mix Up Your Routine

Sticking to the same routine for too long can lead to boredom and plateaus. It's important to keep workouts fresh and challenging by mixing things up regularly.
How to Switch Things Up:

- **Change the exercises:** Rotate new exercises into your routine every few weeks. Try different variations of your go-to moves or incorporate new body parts.
- **Alternate workout styles:** Switch between circuit training, high-intensity interval training (HIIT), and strength-focused sessions. This not only keeps things interesting but also challenges your body in different ways.
- **Add a challenge day:** Dedicate one day a week to trying something new or testing your limits. For example, try an all-cardio day, a bodyweight endurance challenge, or a time

trial for how many squats or push-ups you can do in 5 minutes.

Overcoming Common Challenges and Staying Consistent

Even with the best intentions, there will be days when sticking to your workout routine feels tough. Whether it's due to a busy schedule, lack of motivation, or feeling too tired. You can expect obstacles, in all shapes and sizes; it's just a part of life. Here's how to tackle some of the more common ones and stay on track.

Lack of Time

One of the biggest hurdles for many people is finding time to exercise, especially with work, family, and other responsibilities. But, remember, even short workouts can be effective if done consistently.

Tips for Finding Time:

- **Break it up:** If you can't find a clear 30 minutes all at once, break your workout into shorter 10 or 15 minute sessions spread throughout the day. A quick morning session and another during lunch or at night before bed still add up.
- **Use "found" time:** Sneak in mini workouts during idle moments, like doing squats while you wait for the kettle to boil or a quick plank during a TV commercial break.
- **Prioritize it:** Block off your workout time in your calendar just like you would a work meeting or an appointment. It's time for your health and well being- don't skip it.

Low Motivation

There will be days when your motivation is low, and that's

completely normal. The key is to have strategies in place to keep you moving, even when you don't feel like it.

Motivation Boosters:

- **Set small, immediate goals:** Instead of focusing on the long-term goal, set a tiny goal for the day, like "I'll just do 5 minutes" or "I'll just start with a warm-up." Often, once you start moving, you'll feel more motivated to continue.
- **Use reminders:** Post motivational quotes, put your workout gear out the night before, or set reminders on your phone to nudge you into action.
- **Find accountability:** Share your goals with a friend or workout partner, or even post your progress on social media. Knowing someone is rooting for you or checking in can be a powerful motivator.

Feeling Too Tired

After a long day, the last thing you might want to do is exercise, but movement can actually help boost your energy levels. It's all about getting started.

Tips for Exercising When Tired:

- **Do a short workout:** Even 10-15 minutes of light movement can help wake you up and improve your mood. You don't need to go full intensity- just get moving.
- **Choose easy exercise:** On low-energy days, focus on simple exercises like walking, stretching, or yoga. These movements help you stay active without exhausting you further.
- **Listen to your body:** If you're genuinely too tired or feeling burnt out, it's okay to take a rest day. Just make sure to get back into your routine the next day.

Not Seeing Immediate Results

Fitness progress doesn't always happen as quickly as we'd like and it's easy to feel discouraged when you don't see immediate physical changes. But, keep in mind that consistency is key and results WILL come with time.

How to Stay Patient:

- **Focus on non-scale victories:** Progress isn't just about weight loss or muscle gain. Pay attention to other improvements, like increased energy, better mood, better sleep, or how much easier exercises are getting.
- **Celebrate small wins:** Even completing your workout when you don't feel like it is a victory. Celebrate these moments; they are the building blocks of long-term success.
- **Trust the process:** Results come with time and consistency. Don't give up just because you haven't hit your goal yet. Keep going and the changes will come.

Dealing with Plateaus

Hitting a plateau is when you stop seeing progress, even though you're sticking to your routine. This is a common experience, but it can be frustrating. The key is to change things up.

Tips for Breaking Through Plateaus:

- **Switch up your routine:** Try new exercises, increase the intensity, or add new equipment to challenge your muscles in different ways.
- **Track and adjust:** If you've been doing the same number of reps, sets, or resistance.
- **Rest and recover:** Sometimes, plateaus happen because your body needs more rest. Ensure you're getting enough sleep and taking rest days to allow your muscles to recover and grow stronger.

Managing Injuries or Pain

Injuries or aches can derail your workout routine, but they don't have to stop you completely. It's important to listen to your body and adapt your workouts as needed.

Tips for Dealing with Injuries:

- **Focus on recovery:** If you're injured, prioritize healing first. Gentle stretches, mobility work, or light exercises that don't aggravate the injury can help you stay active while recovering.
- **Modify exercises:** You may need to switch to lower-impact exercises, like walking, swimming, or cycling, that are gentler on your body. Modify your regular workouts to avoid putting stress on the injured area.
- **Consult a professional:** If the pain persists, consult a physical therapist or fitness professional who can help guide you on how to safely continue exercising.

Nutrition Basics for Beginners

While exercise is a crucial part of any fitness journey, nutrition plays an equally important role in achieving your health and fitness goals. Eating well helps you recover from workouts, boosts energy, and supports overall well-being. Here are some essential nutrition tips to help you get started.

Understanding Macronutrients

Macronutrients are the nutrients your body needs in larger amounts to function properly. They include carbohydrates, proteins, and fats. Understanding these can help you make healthier choices.

- **Carbohydrates:** Commonly called carbs, the body's primary source of energy. Focus on complex carbs like whole grains, fruits, and vegetables, which provide lasting energy and essential nutrients.
- **Proteins:** Essential for muscle repair and growth. Include sources like lean meats, fish, eggs, beans, and nuts in your meals to support your fitness routine.
- **Fats:** Important for hormone production and overall health. Choose healthy fats from sources like avocados, olive oil, nuts and seeds, while limiting saturated and trans fats.

Stay Hydrated

Staying hydrated is vital for overall health and optimal performance during workouts. Water helps regulate body temperature, transports nutrients, and aids digestion.

Tips for Staying Hydrated:

- **Drink water throughout the day:** Aim for at least 8 glasses of water daily, adjusting based on your activity level.
- **Hydrate before, during, and after workouts:** Drink water before your workout to prepare your body, sip water during exercise, and rehydrate afterwards to aid in recovery.
- **Listen to your body:** Thirst is an indicator that your body needs water, so pay attention to it and drink accordingly. Try not to quench your thirst with things that might dehydrate you like coffee, soda, or energy drinks. It's okay to have these things, in moderation, but do not replace water with them.

Eat Balanced Meals

Strive to create balanced meals that include a variety of macronutrients and micronutrients. A well-rounded meal supports energy levels, enhances recovery, and helps maintain a healthy weight.

Components of a Balanced Meal:

- **Protein:** Include a source of protein, i.e. chicken, fish, tofu, or legumes (chickpeas, lentils, black beans, kidney beans, pinto beans, green peas)
- **Carbs:** Add a serving of complex carbohydrates, i.e. brown rice, quinoa, sweet potatoes, whole wheat pasta and bread, barley and oats. Legumes are also a complex carbohydrate.
- **Vegetables:** Fill half your plate with colorful vegetables for vitamins, minerals, and fiber.
- **Healthy fats:** Incorporate healthy fats to enhance satiety, so you feel fuller longer, i.e. olive oil, avocado, nuts, seeds (chia, flax, sunflower, sesame, pumpkin), eggs (especially the yolk).

Practice Portion Control

Portion control is key to maintaining a healthy diet. Eating larger portions than necessary can lead to overeating, while properly managing portion sizes can help you feel satisfied without excess calories.

Tips for Managing Portions:

Use smaller plates: Smaller dishes can help prevent overeating by making portions appear larger.
Listen to your hunger cues: Eat when you're hungry and stop when you are satisfied rather than eating until you're full. Waiting 30 minutes before grabbing another plate, dessert, or a snack can also help.
Plan your meals: Prepare meals in advance to control portion sizes and reduce the temptation to grab unhealthy snacks when you're hungry.

Meal Prep for Success

Meal prepping can save time and help you make healthier choices throughout the week. By preparing your meals in advance, you'll be less likely to reach for convenience foods that may not align with your fitness goals.

Tips for Effective Meal Prep:

Choose a day to prep: Dedicate a specific day, like Sunday, to prepare meals for the week ahead.
Batch cook: Make larger quantities of healthy dishes, such as soups, stews, or grains, and portion them into containers for easy access.
Pack healthy snacks: Prepare grab-and-go snacks like cut-up fruits, veggies with hummus, or homemade energy bars to avoid unhealthy choices when hunger strikes.

Be Mindful of Snacking

Snacking can be part of a healthy diet if done mindfully. Choose nutritious snacks that fuel your body and help maintain energy levels throughout the day.

Healthy Snack Ideas:

- **Fruits:** Fresh fruit like apples, bananas, or berries for quick energy and natural sweetness.
- **Nuts and seeds:** A small handful provides healthy fats and protein, perfect for a satisfying snack.
- **Yogurt:** A serving of yogurt (preferably Greek) topped with fruits or a sprinkle of granola for added texture and nutrients.
- **Veggies and dip:** Raw veggies like carrots or bell peppers with hummus or guacamole for a crunchy, satisfying snack.

Listen to Your Body

Ultimately, your body knows what it needs. Pay attention to how different foods make you feel and adjust your diet accordingly. Eating should be an enjoyable experience, so find what works for you and makes you feel your best.

Tips:

- **Enjoy your meals:** Take time to savor your food, take small bites and don't race through your meal. This can enhance your satisfaction and help you recognize when you're full.
- **Experiment with flavors:** Try new recipes and ingredients to discover what you enjoy and find ways to make healthy eating fun.
- **Reflect on your choices:** After meals, take a moment to assess how you feel. Are you satisfied? Energized? Adjust your meals based on your reflections.

Resources and Tools for Success

While I aimed to include most everything a beginner would need to become fit in this book, some other resources or tools can significantly enhance your fitness journey or help you through a rough patch. This section includes helpful apps, websites, and additional resources to support your efforts.

Fitness Apps

Using fitness apps can help you track workouts, monitor progress, and stay motivated. Here are some popular options:

- **MyFitnessPal:** Great for tracking nutrition, workouts, and overall progress. Its extensive food database makes it easy to log meals.
- **Nike Training Club:** Offers a variety of guided workouts for all fitness levels, with options for bodyweight exercises and those using minimal equipment.
- **Fitbod:** Tailors workouts based on your fitness level and available equipment, making it easy to plan and adapt your routine.
- **Seven:** Focused on quick, 7-minute workouts, this app is perfect for busy schedules and encourages consistency.

Online Workout Platforms

Many online platforms provide guided workout videos and training programs, allowing you to exercise at home. Here are some popular choices:

- **YouTube:** A variety of channels offer free workout videos for all fitness levels.

- **Beachbody On Demand:** Subscription-based service that provides access to various workout programs, including yoga, strength training, and high-intensity workouts.
- **Peloton App:** While known for its cycling classes, the Peloton app also includes strength, yoga, and meditation classes that can be accessed without a bike.

Websites and Blogs

Several websites and blogs offer valuable fitness information, tips, and resources. Consider exploring these:

- **ACE Fitness:** Provides a wealth of articles, workout plans, and resources for all fitness levels, written by certified fitness professionals.
- **Nerd Fitness:** A unique take on fitness, combining geek culture and wellness advice to create a supportive community for all fitness levels.
- **The Fitnessista:** Offers healthy recipes, workout ideas, and lifestyle tips, particularly for busy moms.

Nutrition Resources

Complementing your workouts with proper nutrition is essential for overall health. Consider these resources for meal planning and healthy eating:

- **Eat This, Not That!:** A website and book series that help you make healthier food choices while dining out or shopping for groceries.
- **Forks Over Knives:** Offers a wide range of plant-based recipes, meal plans, and tips for incorporating more whole foods into your diet.
- **Nutrition.gov:** A government resource providing reliable nutrition information, healthy eating tips, and meal planning resources.

Community and Support

Finding a supportive community can help keep you motivated and accountable. Here are some ways to connect with others on similar journeys:

- **Join Local Fitness Classes:** Participating in local classes, such as yoga, Zumba, or boot camps, can help you meet like-minded individuals.
- **Online Forums:** Websites like Reddit (e.g., r/fitness) and fitness-focused Facebook groups provide platforms for discussion, support, and motivation.
- **Challenges and Events:** Consider participating in local fitness challenges, charity walks, or virtual races to connect with others and stay motivated.

Books and Guides

Reading books on fitness, nutrition, and wellness can provide valuable insights and motivation. Here are a few recommended reads.

"The Fitness Mindset" by Brian Keane: This book explores the psychological aspect of fitness, providing tips for building a positive mindset and staying committed to your goals.

"How Not to Die" by Dr. Michael Greger: A comprehensive guide on the impact of nutrition on health and how to incorporate more plant-based foods into your diet.

"Body Boss" by Tiffiny Hall: Offers a unique approach to fitness and nutrition, focusing on both physical and mental well-being.

Final Thoughts

Congratulations on taking the first steps toward a healthier, more active lifestyle! Your commitment to incorporating exercise into your daily routine is a significant achievement and every effort you make counts. Remember that fitness is not just a destination; it's a lifelong commitment to caring for your body and mind.

Embrace the Journey

Fitness is a personal journey and each person's path is unique. Embrace where you are today and celebrate every small victory along the way. Whether it's completing your first workout, increasing your reps, or simply feeling more energetic, every achievement matters.

Be Patient with Yourself

Progress takes time and it's essential to be patient with yourself as you adapt to new habits. Of course there will be ups and downs, but don't get discouraged. Consistency is key and every step you take brings you closer to your goals. Remember that it's okay to have setbacks- what matters is how you respond and keep moving forward.

Keep Learning and Growing

As you continue your fitness journey, be open to learning and exploring new things. Try different workout styles, experiment with healthy recipes, and seek out resources that resonate with you. The more you learn, the more empowered you'll feel to make choices that support your health and well-being.

Find Your Support System

Surround yourself with supportive individuals who uplift and motivate you. Whether it's friends, family, or an online community, having people to share your journey with can make all the difference. Don't hesitate to reach out for encouragement or advice and remember that you're not alone in this process.

Celebrate Your Achievements

Take time to acknowledge your hard work and progress. Celebrate your milestones, no matter how small, and reflect on how far you've come. Consider keeping a journal of your achievements, both big and small, as a reminder of your dedication and growth.

Stay Committed to Your Goals

Commitment is a crucial factor in achieving your fitness goals. Set realistic, meaningful goals that resonate with you and revisit them regularly to stay focused. Remember, it's not about perfection- it's about progress. As you move forward, keep in mind that the journey to health and fitness is as rewarding as the destination. Enjoy the process, be kind to yourself, and keep striving for balance in all areas of your life.

Thank you for allowing this book to be a part of that and here's to a healthier, happier you!

Glossary of Terms

Active Recovery: Light physical activity performed on rest days, such as walking or gentle yoga, aimed at promoting blood flow and recovery without intense exertion.

BMI (Body Mass Index): A numerical value derived from height and weight, used as a general indicator of body composition and health. However, it doesn't account for muscle mass or distribution.

Bodyweight Exercises: Exercises that use the weight of your own body as resistance, requiring no additional equipment (e.g., push-ups, squats, lunges).

Circuit Training: A workout style that involves performing a series of exercises in sequence, with minimal rest in between. Circuit training can improve strength and cardiovascular fitness.

Compound Exercises: Exercises that engage multiple muscle groups at once, such as squats, deadlifts, and bench presses. These are often more efficient for building strength.

Cool Down: A period of low-intensity exercise or stretching following a workout, aimed at gradually lowering heart rate and aiding recovery.

Core: Refers to the muscles in your abdomen, lower back, hips, and pelvis. A strong core is essential for stability and overall functional fitness.

Endurance: The ability to sustain physical activity over an extended period. Cardiovascular endurance is crucial for activities like running, cycling, and swimming.

Flexibility: The ability of a muscle or joint to move through its full range of motion. Flexibility exercises, such as stretching, help improve mobility and reduce the risk of injury.

HIIT (High-Intensity Interval Training): A workout style that alternates between short bursts of intense activity and periods of rest or lower-intensity exercises. HIIT is effective for improving cardiovascular fitness and burning calories.

Isometric Exercises: Exercises that involve holding a position or contraction without changing the length of the muscle, such as planks or wall sits.

Macronutrients: Nutrients that provide energy, including carbohydrates, proteins, and fats. Each plays a different role in the body and is essential for overall health.

Metabolism: The process by which your body converts food into energy. A higher metabolic rate can aid in weight loss and overall energy levels.

Micro-nutrients: Vitamins and minerals that are crucial for overall health but are needed in smaller amounts compared to macronutrients. They support various bodily functions.

Plyometrics: Exercises that involve explosive movements, such as jump squats or box jumps, aimed at improving power and athletic performance.

Resistance Bands: Elastic bands used for strength training, available in various resistance levels. They are versatile and portable, making them ideal for home workouts.

Reps (Repetitions): The number of times you perform a specific exercise or movement in a row. For example, doing 10 push-ups means completing 10 reps.

Rest Day: A day dedicated to recovery and avoiding intense physical activity. Rest days are essential for muscle recovery and preventing overtraining.

Sets: A group of consecutive repetitions of an exercise. For example, if you do 10 push-ups and then take a break, that constitutes one set of 10 reps.

Warm-Up: A series of light exercises or stretches performed before a workout to prepare the body for physical activity and reduce the risk of injury.

www.ingramcontent.com/pod-product-compliance
Lightning Source LLC
Chambersburg PA
CBHW031425250726
48656CB00002B/837

* 9 7 9 8 3 0 3 9 3 5 1 1 2 *